Table of Contents

Table of Contents

Page #   Recipe / Description

Table of Contents

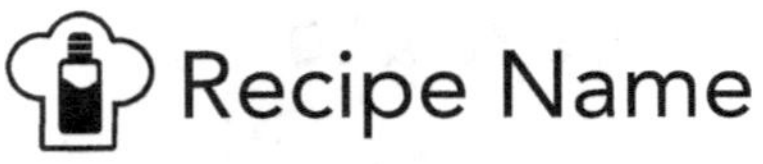 # Recipe Name

 Rating

☆ ☆ ☆ ☆ ☆

Ingredients

Directions

Uses & Notes

1

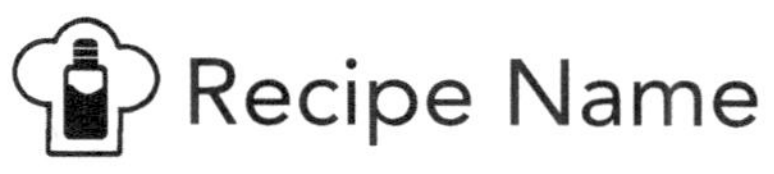 # Recipe Name

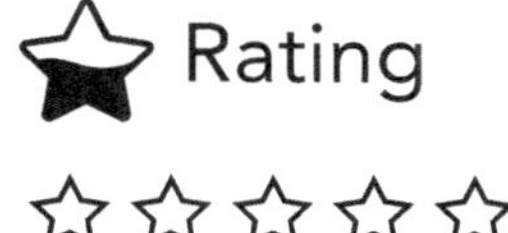 Rating

☆ ☆ ☆ ☆ ☆

Ingredients

Directions

Uses & Notes

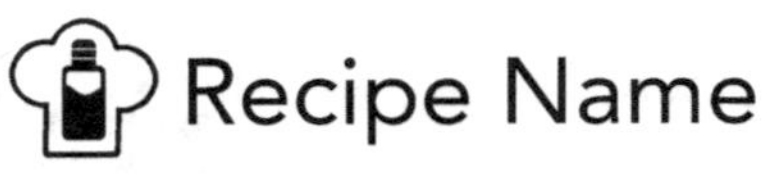 # Recipe Name

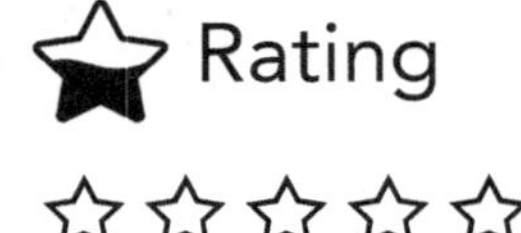 Rating

☆ ☆ ☆ ☆ ☆

Ingredients

Directions

Uses & Notes

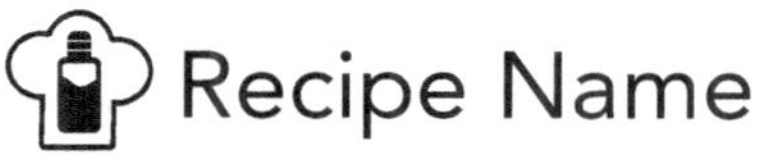 # Recipe Name

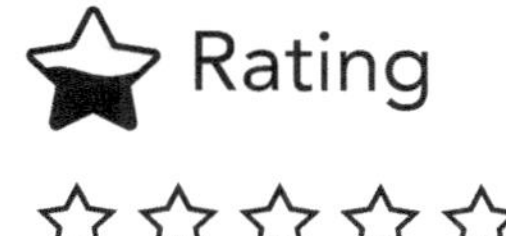 Rating

☆ ☆ ☆ ☆ ☆

Ingredients

Directions

Uses & Notes

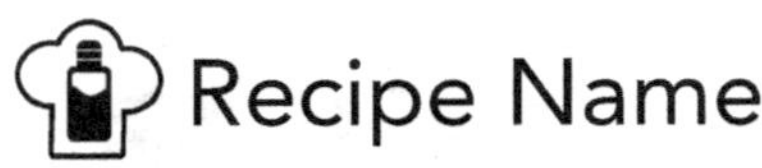 **Recipe Name**

Rating
☆ ☆ ☆ ☆ ☆

Ingredients

Directions

Uses & Notes

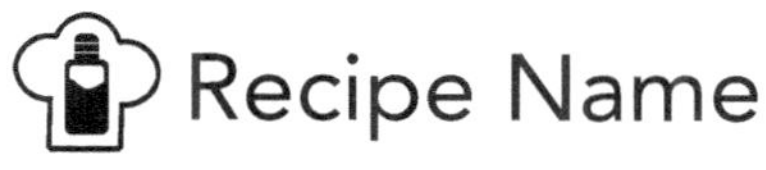 Recipe Name

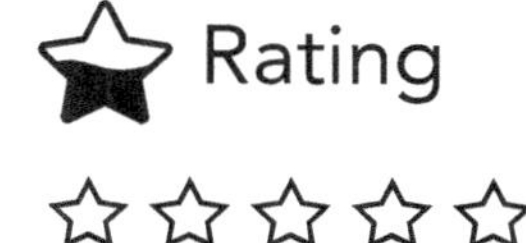 Rating

☆ ☆ ☆ ☆ ☆

Ingredients

Directions

Uses & Notes

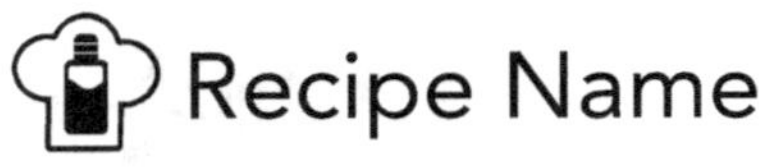 Recipe Name

 Rating

☆ ☆ ☆ ☆ ☆

Ingredients

Directions

Uses & Notes

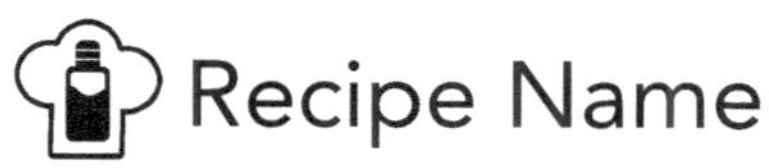 # Recipe Name

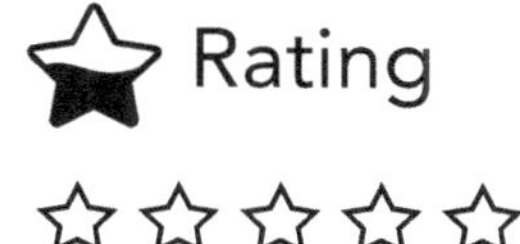 Rating

☆ ☆ ☆ ☆ ☆

Ingredients

Directions

Uses & Notes

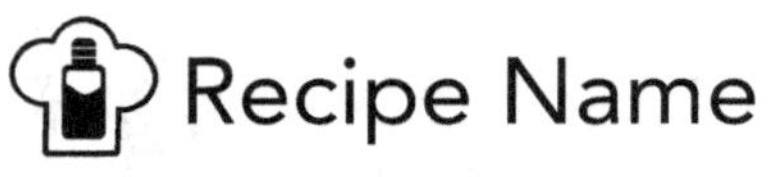 # Recipe Name

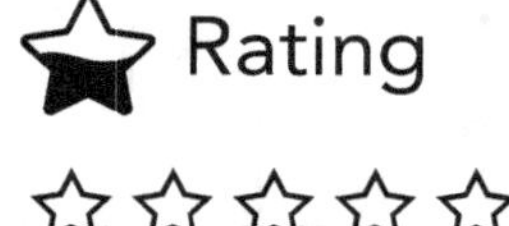 Rating
☆ ☆ ☆ ☆ ☆

Ingredients

Directions

Uses & Notes

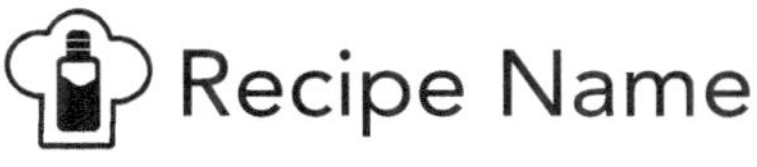 # Recipe Name

Rating

☆ ☆ ☆ ☆ ☆

Ingredients

Directions

Uses & Notes

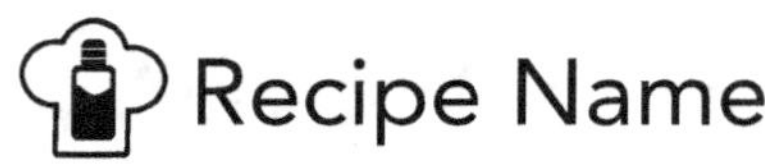 Recipe Name

Rating

☆ ☆ ☆ ☆ ☆

Ingredients

Directions

Uses & Notes

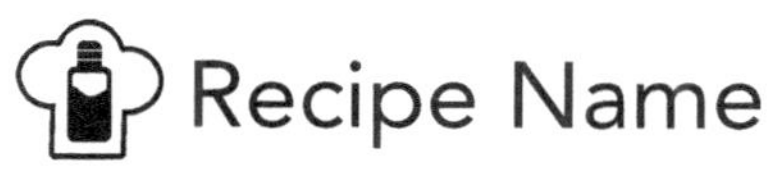 # Recipe Name

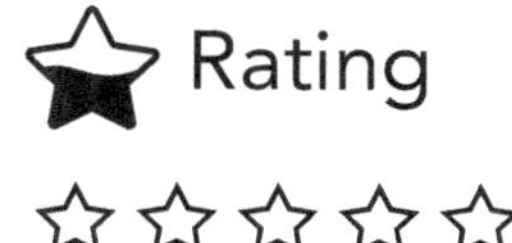

Rating

☆ ☆ ☆ ☆ ☆

Ingredients

Directions

Uses & Notes

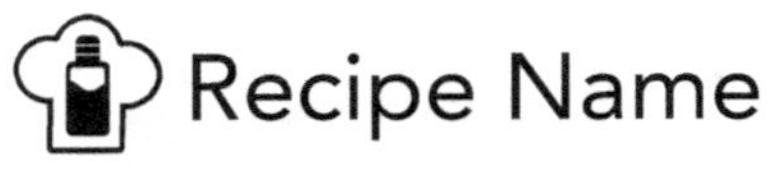 **Recipe Name**

⭐ Rating
☆ ☆ ☆ ☆ ☆

Ingredients

Directions

Uses & Notes

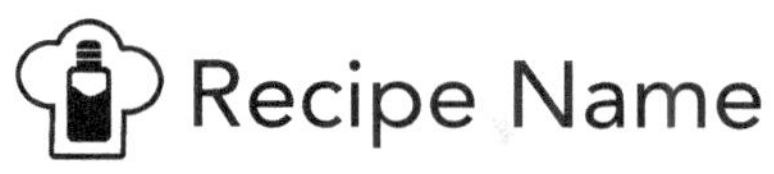 # Recipe Name

 Rating

☆ ☆ ☆ ☆ ☆

Ingredients

Directions

Uses & Notes

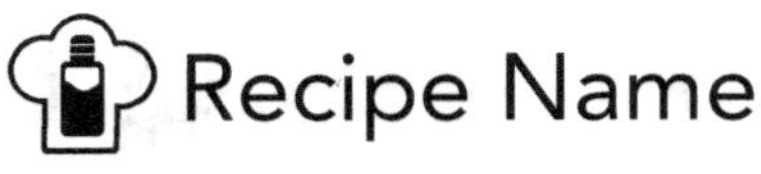 Recipe Name 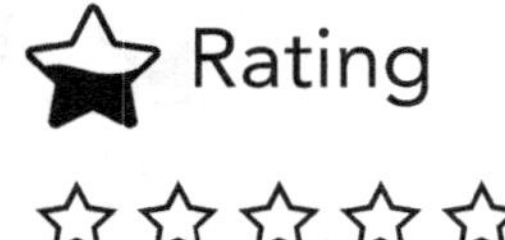 Rating

☆ ☆ ☆ ☆ ☆

Ingredients

Directions

Uses & Notes

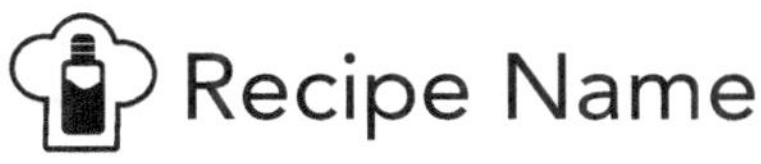 # Recipe Name

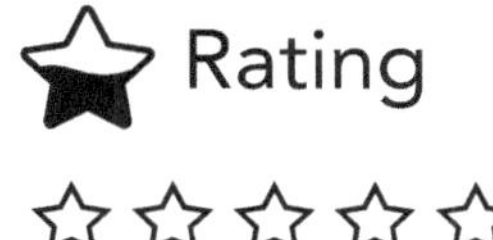 Rating

☆ ☆ ☆ ☆ ☆

Ingredients

Directions

Uses & Notes

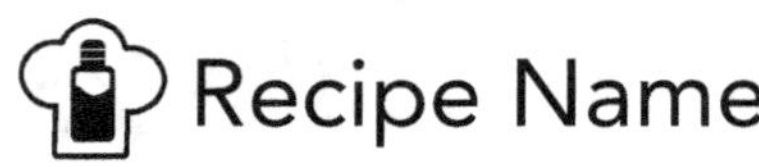 # Recipe Name

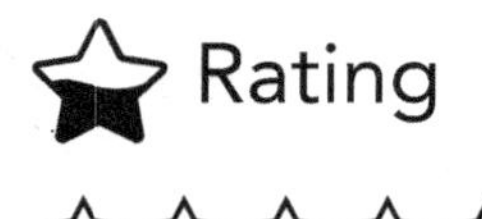 Rating

☆ ☆ ☆ ☆ ☆

Ingredients

Directions

Uses & Notes

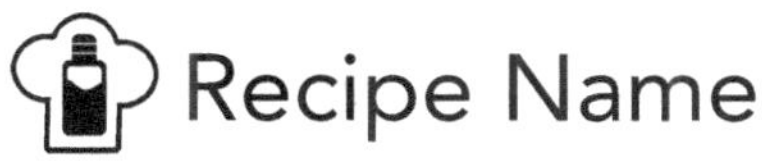 # Recipe Name

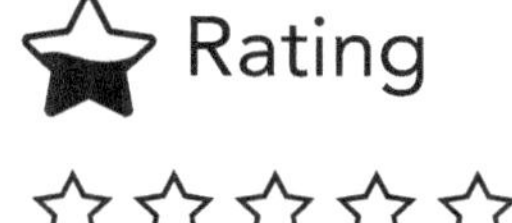 Rating

☆ ☆ ☆ ☆ ☆

Ingredients

Directions

Uses & Notes

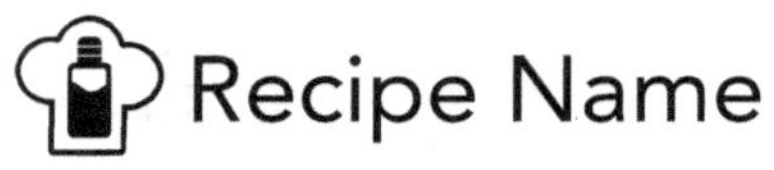 Recipe Name

Rating

☆ ☆ ☆ ☆ ☆

Ingredients

Directions

Uses & Notes

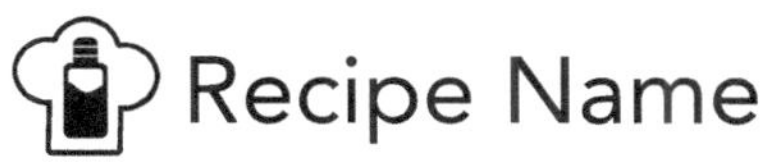 # Recipe Name

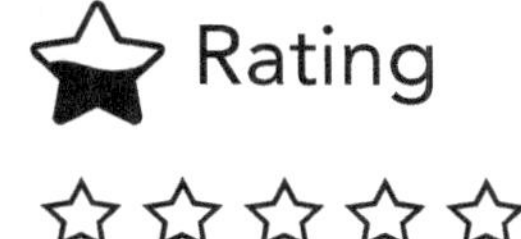 Rating

☆ ☆ ☆ ☆ ☆

Ingredients

Directions

Uses & Notes

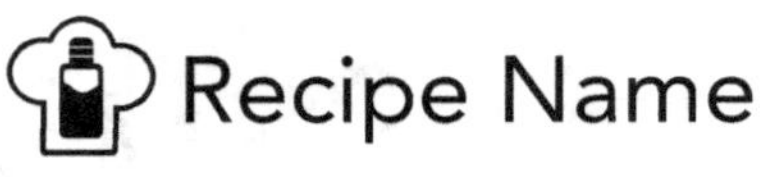 Recipe Name

Rating

☆ ☆ ☆ ☆ ☆

Ingredients

Directions

Uses & Notes

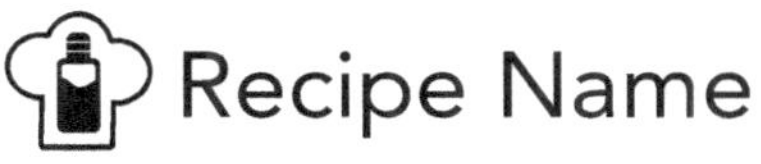 **Recipe Name**

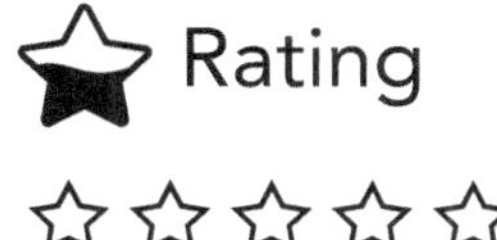 Rating
☆ ☆ ☆ ☆ ☆

Ingredients

Directions

Uses & Notes

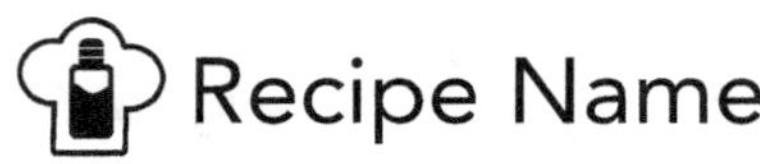 # Recipe Name

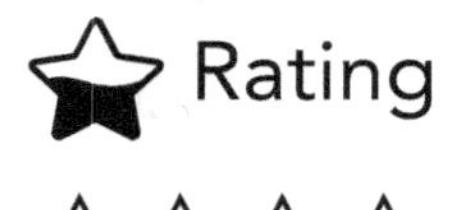 Rating

☆ ☆ ☆ ☆ ☆

Ingredients

Directions

Uses & Notes

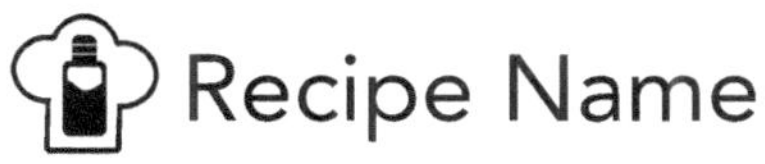 # Recipe Name

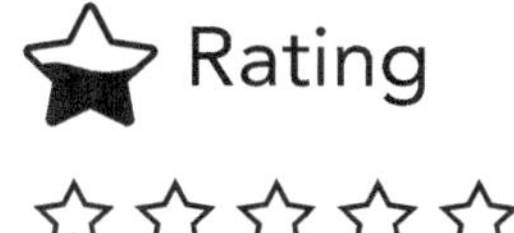 Rating

☆ ☆ ☆ ☆ ☆

Ingredients

Directions

Uses & Notes

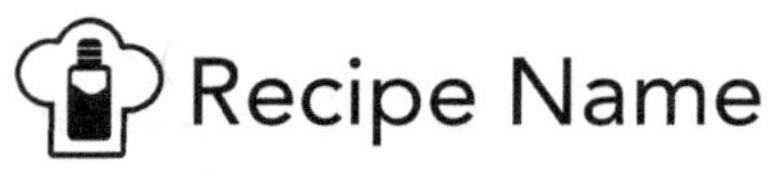 # Recipe Name

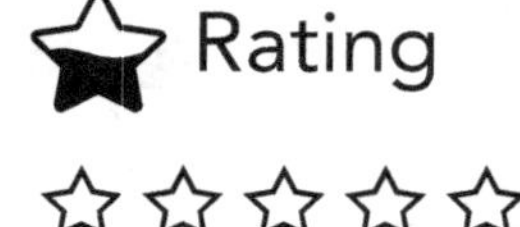 Rating

☆ ☆ ☆ ☆ ☆

Ingredients

Directions

Uses & Notes

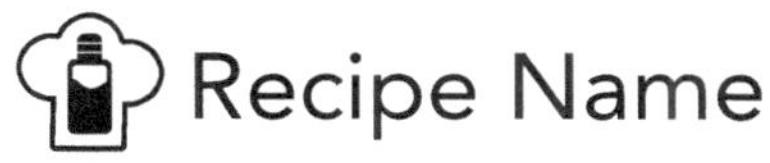 **Recipe Name**

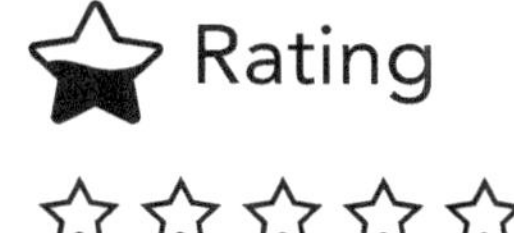 **Rating**

☆ ☆ ☆ ☆ ☆

Ingredients

Directions

Uses & Notes

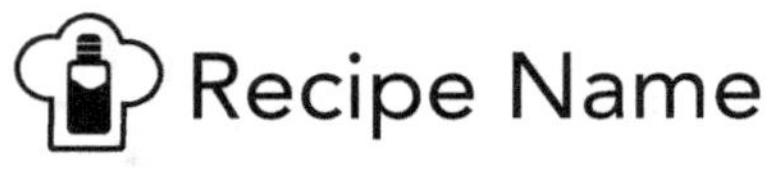 Recipe Name

Rating
☆ ☆ ☆ ☆ ☆

Ingredients

Directions

Uses & Notes

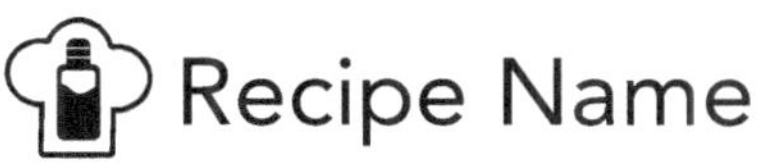 # Recipe Name

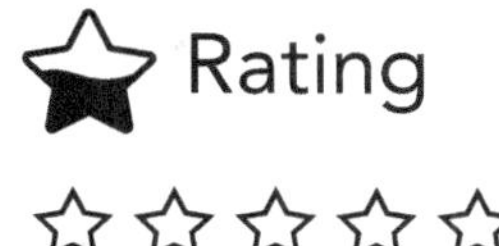

____

Ingredients

Directions

Uses & Notes

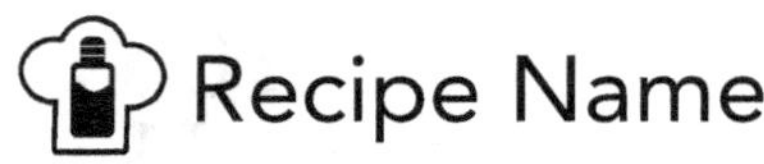 Recipe Name

☆ Rating
☆ ☆ ☆ ☆ ☆

Ingredients

_______________________ _______________________

_______________________ _______________________

_______________________ _______________________

_______________________ _______________________

_______________________ _______________________

Directions

____

____

____

____

____

____

Uses & Notes

____

____

____

____

____

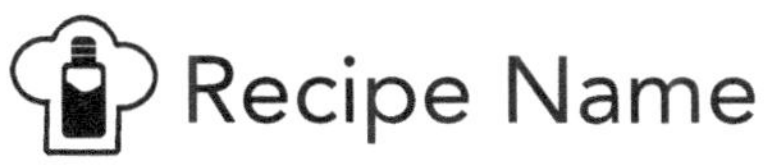 # Recipe Name

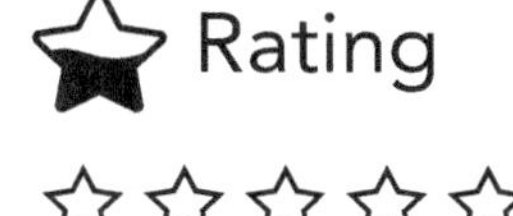

Rating

☆ ☆ ☆ ☆ ☆

Ingredients

Directions

Uses & Notes

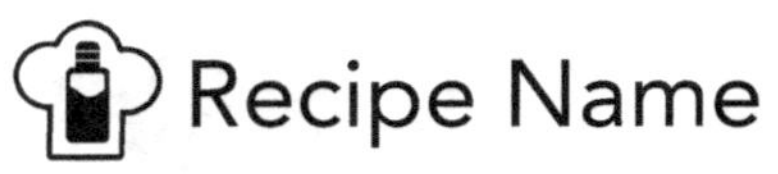 # Recipe Name

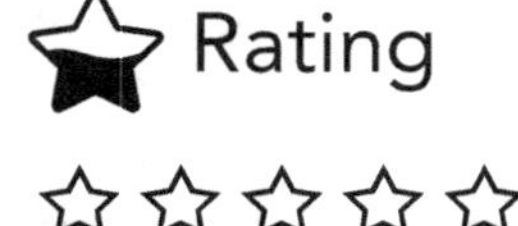 Rating

☆ ☆ ☆ ☆ ☆

Ingredients

Directions

Uses & Notes

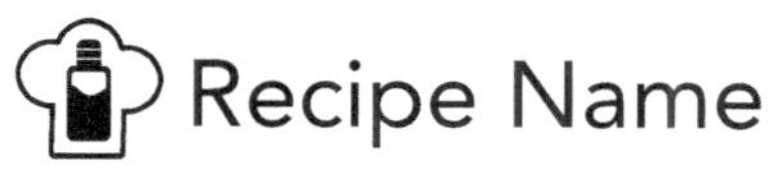 # Recipe Name

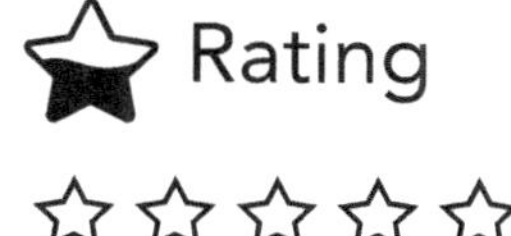 Rating

☆ ☆ ☆ ☆ ☆

Ingredients

Directions

Uses & Notes

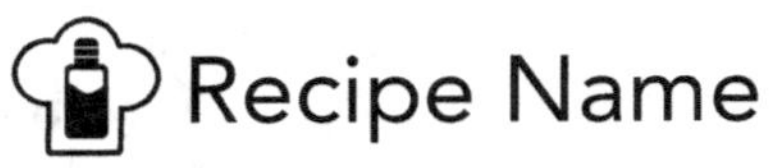 # Recipe Name

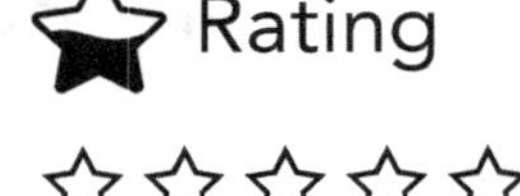 Rating

☆ ☆ ☆ ☆ ☆

Ingredients

Directions

Uses & Notes

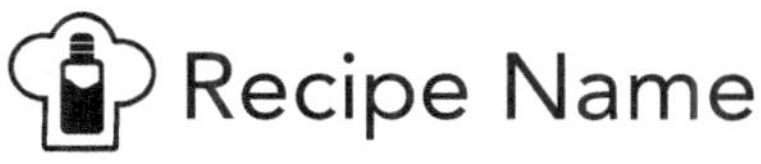 # Recipe Name

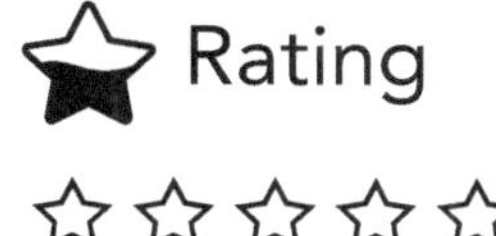 Rating

☆ ☆ ☆ ☆ ☆

Ingredients

Directions

Uses & Notes

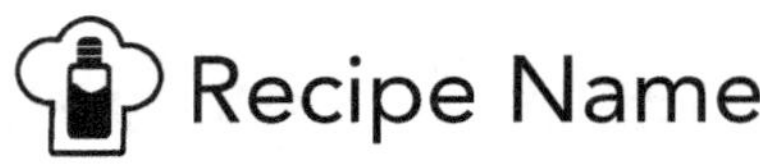 # Recipe Name

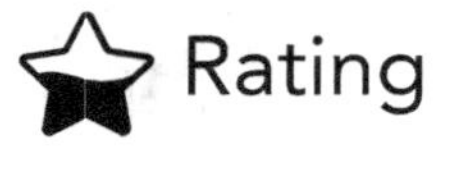 Rating

☆ ☆ ☆ ☆ ☆

Ingredients

Directions

Uses & Notes

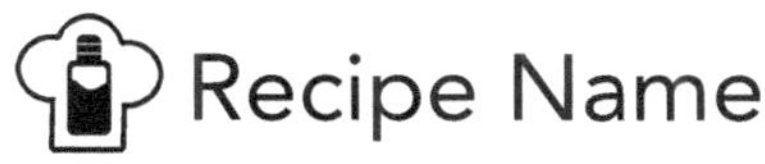 # Recipe Name

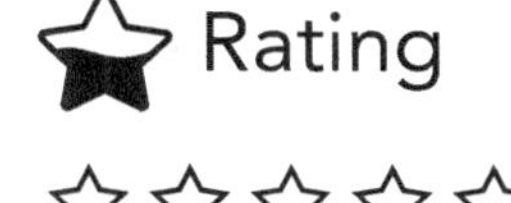 Rating

☆ ☆ ☆ ☆ ☆

Ingredients

Directions

Uses & Notes

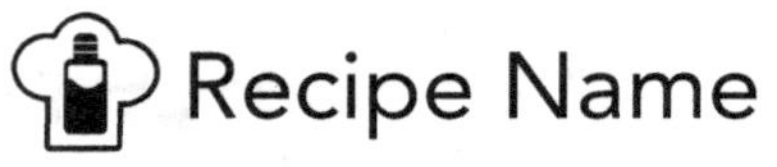 Recipe Name

Rating

☆ ☆ ☆ ☆ ☆

Ingredients

Directions

Uses & Notes

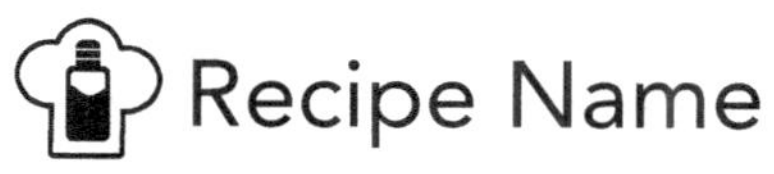 # Recipe Name

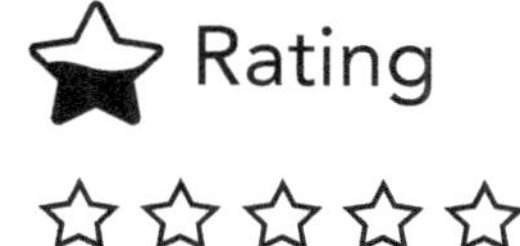 Rating

☆ ☆ ☆ ☆ ☆

Ingredients

_______________________   _______________________
_______________________   _______________________
_______________________   _______________________
_______________________   _______________________
_______________________   _______________________

Directions

____
____
____
____
____

Uses & Notes

____
____
____
____
____

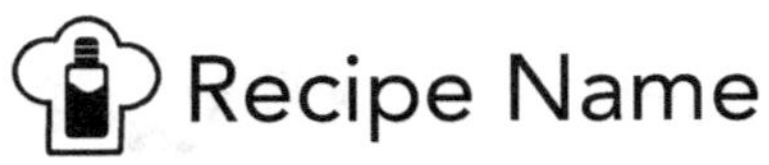 # Recipe Name

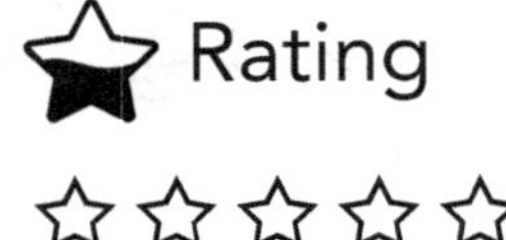 Rating

☆ ☆ ☆ ☆ ☆

Ingredients

Directions

Uses & Notes

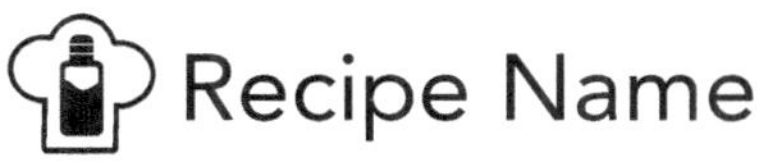 # Recipe Name

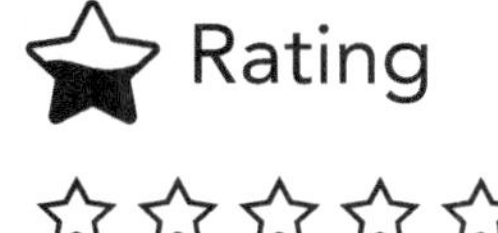 Rating

☆ ☆ ☆ ☆ ☆

Ingredients

Directions

Uses & Notes

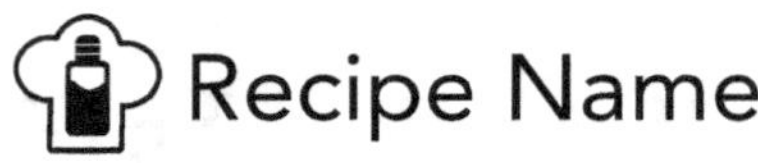 Recipe Name

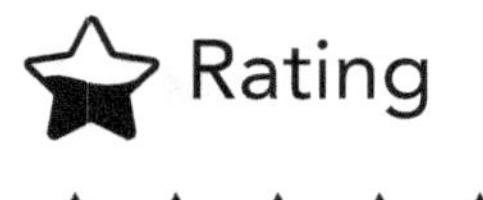 Rating

☆ ☆ ☆ ☆ ☆

Ingredients

Directions

Uses & Notes

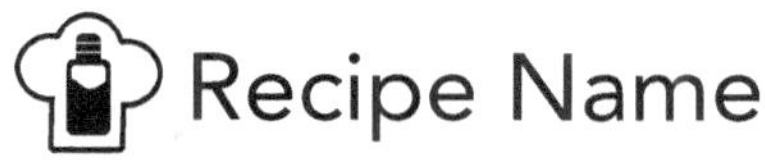 # Recipe Name

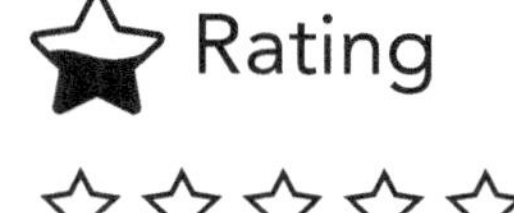 Rating

☆ ☆ ☆ ☆ ☆

Ingredients

Directions

Uses & Notes

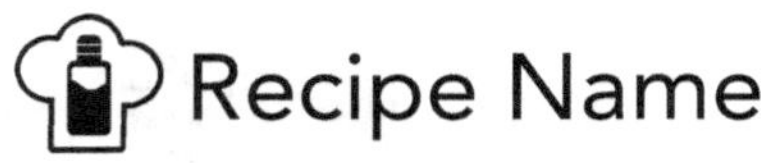 **Recipe Name**

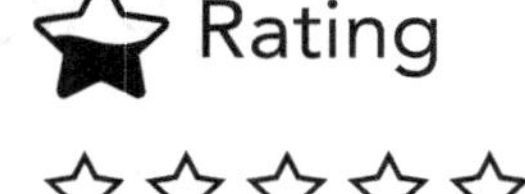

Rating

☆ ☆ ☆ ☆ ☆

Ingredients

Directions

Uses & Notes

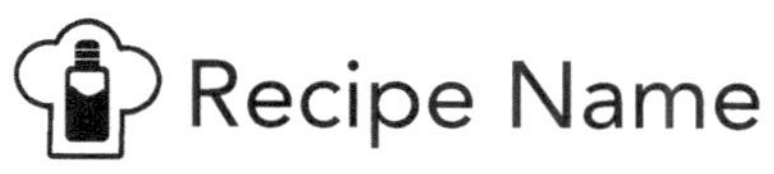 # Recipe Name

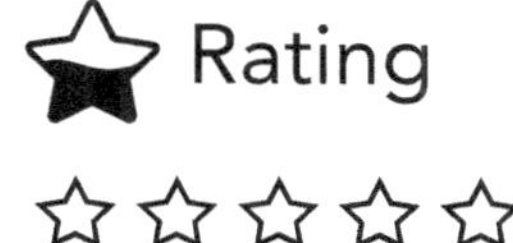 Rating
☆ ☆ ☆ ☆ ☆

Ingredients

Directions

Uses & Notes

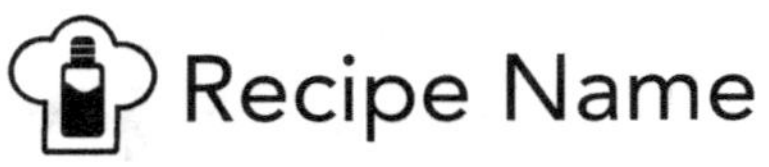 **Recipe Name**

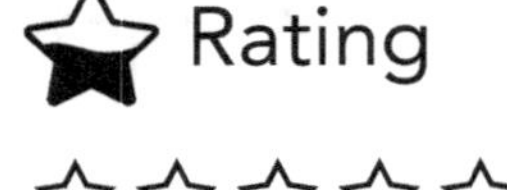 Rating
☆ ☆ ☆ ☆ ☆

Ingredients

Directions

Uses & Notes

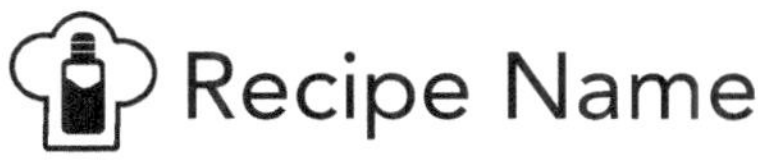 # Recipe Name

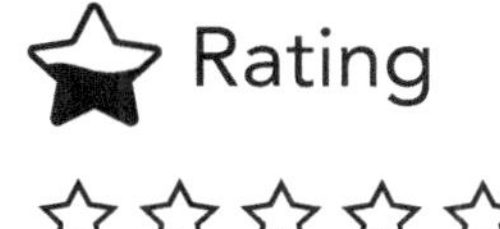 Rating

☆ ☆ ☆ ☆ ☆

Ingredients

Directions

Uses & Notes

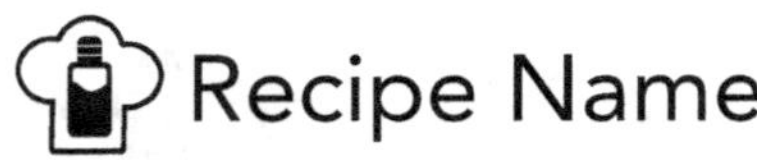 # Recipe Name

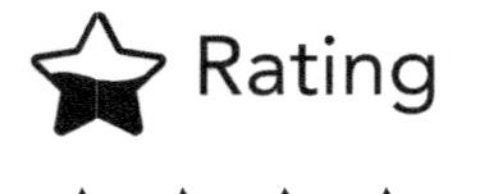 Rating

☆ ☆ ☆ ☆ ☆

Ingredients

Directions

Uses & Notes

Ingredients

Directions

Uses & Notes

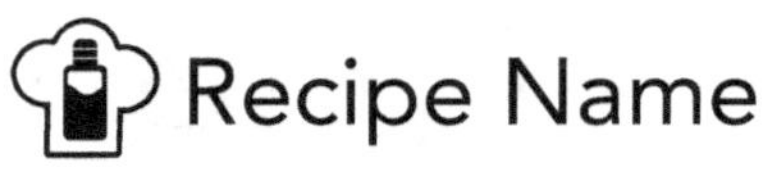 **Recipe Name**

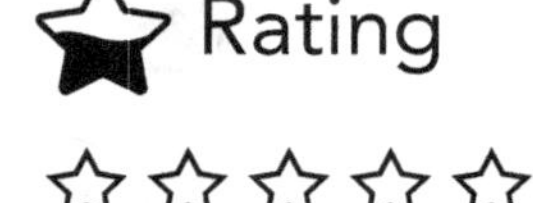 **Rating**

☆ ☆ ☆ ☆ ☆

Ingredients

Directions

Uses & Notes

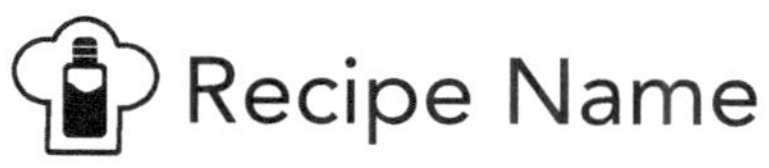 # Recipe Name

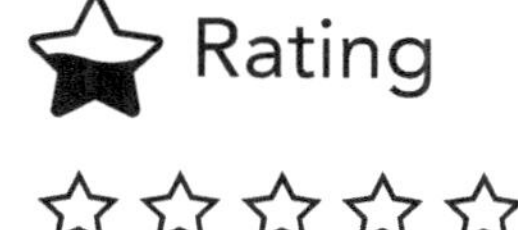 Rating

☆ ☆ ☆ ☆ ☆

Ingredients

Directions

Uses & Notes

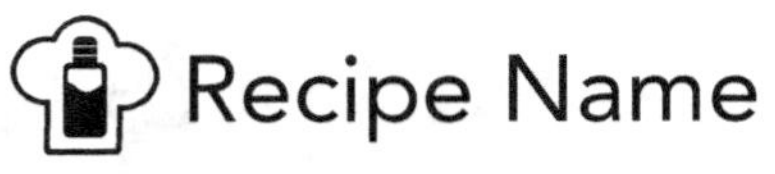 **Recipe Name**

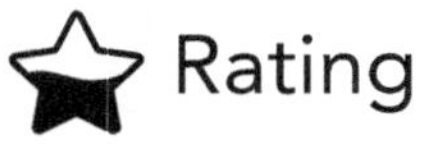 **Rating**
☆ ☆ ☆ ☆ ☆

Ingredients

Directions

Uses & Notes

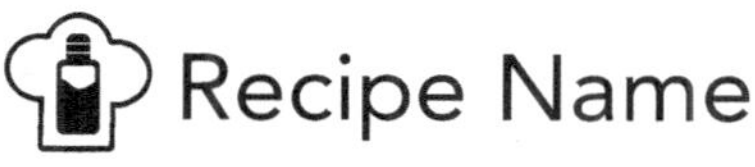 # Recipe Name

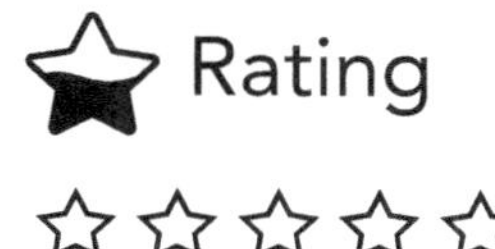 Rating

☆ ☆ ☆ ☆ ☆

Ingredients

Directions

Uses & Notes

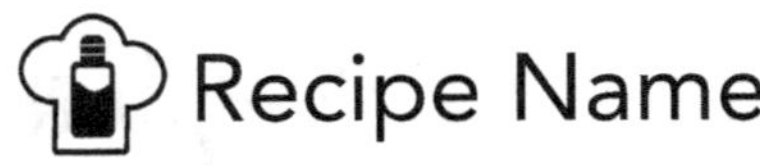 # Recipe Name

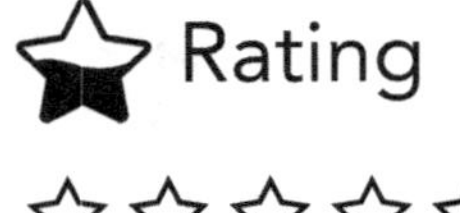 Rating

☆ ☆ ☆ ☆ ☆

Ingredients

Directions

Uses & Notes

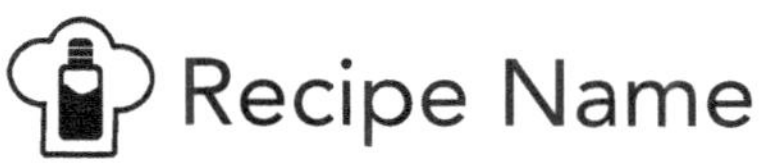 # Recipe Name

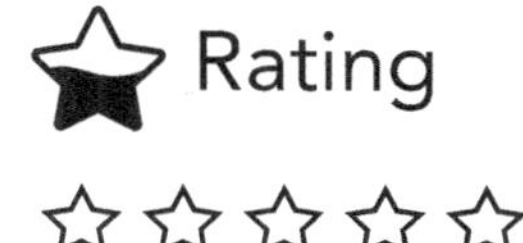 Rating

☆ ☆ ☆ ☆ ☆

Ingredients

Directions

Uses & Notes

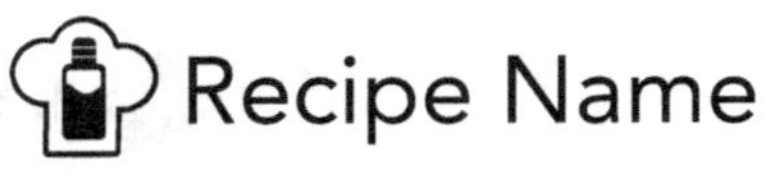 **Recipe Name**

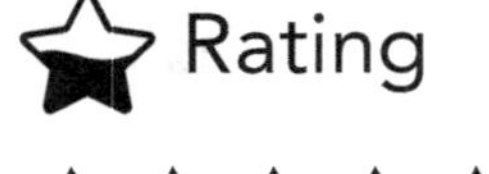 **Rating**

☆ ☆ ☆ ☆ ☆

Ingredients

Directions

Uses & Notes

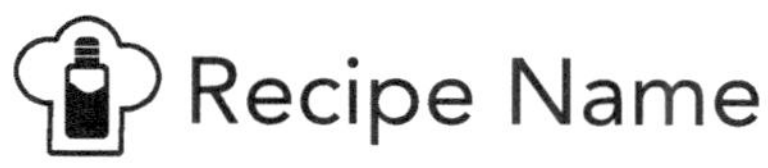 # Recipe Name

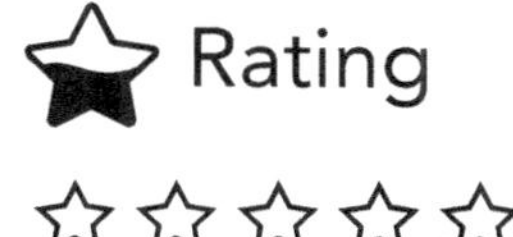
Rating
☆ ☆ ☆ ☆ ☆

Ingredients

Directions

Uses & Notes

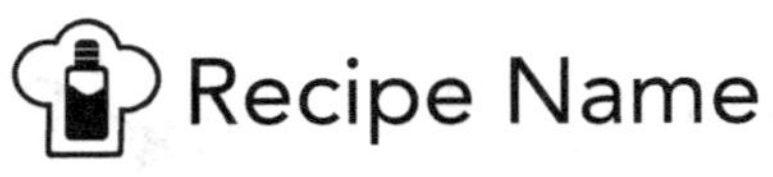 **Recipe Name**

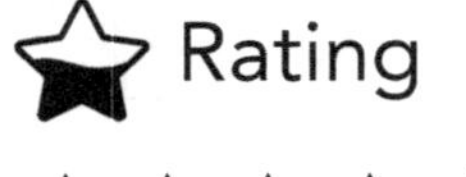 **Rating**

☆ ☆ ☆ ☆ ☆

Ingredients

Directions

Uses & Notes

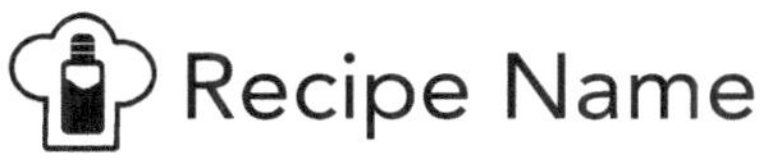 # Recipe Name

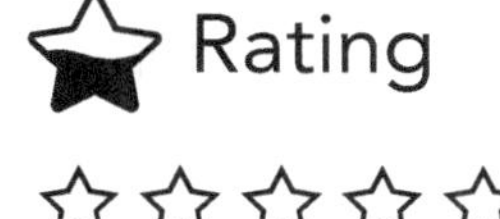

Rating

☆ ☆ ☆ ☆ ☆

Ingredients

Directions

Uses & Notes

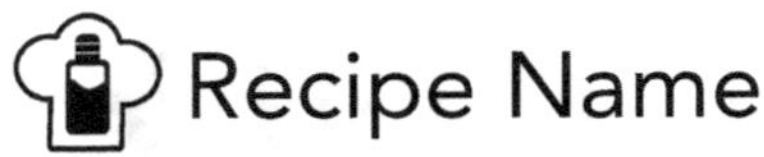 **Recipe Name**

Rating

☆ ☆ ☆ ☆ ☆

Ingredients

Directions

Uses & Notes

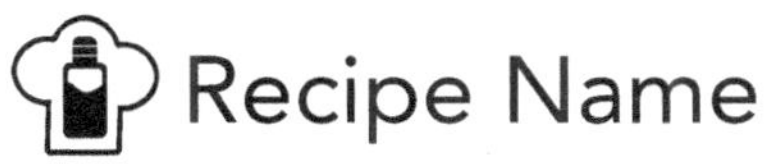 # Recipe Name

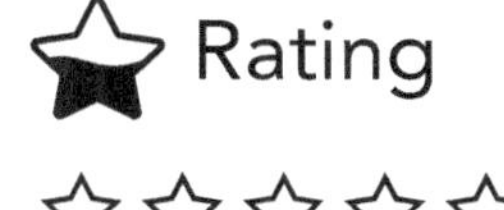 Rating

☆ ☆ ☆ ☆ ☆

Ingredients

Directions

Uses & Notes

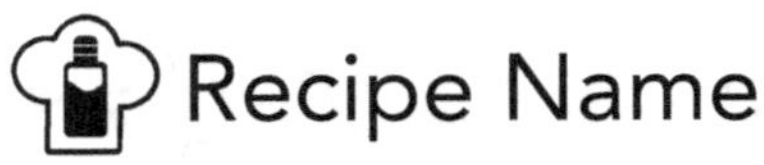 # Recipe Name

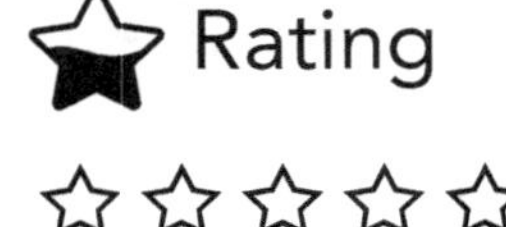 Rating

☆ ☆ ☆ ☆ ☆

Ingredients

Directions

Uses & Notes

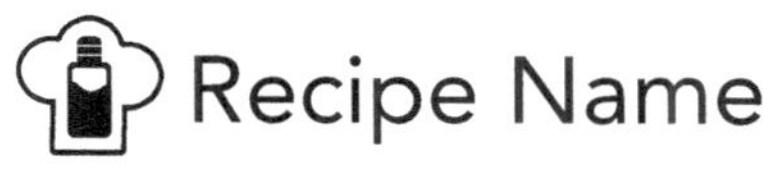 # Recipe Name

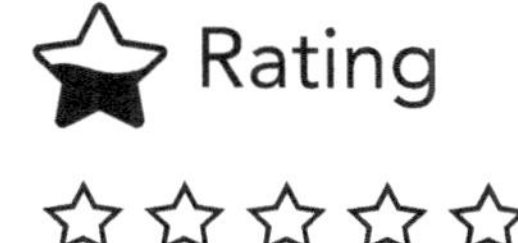 Rating
☆ ☆ ☆ ☆ ☆

Ingredients

Directions

Uses & Notes

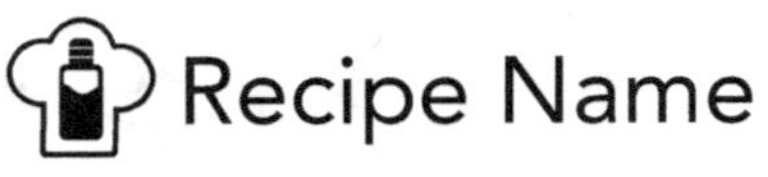 # Recipe Name

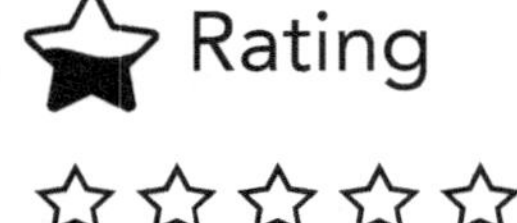 Rating

☆ ☆ ☆ ☆ ☆

Ingredients

Directions

Uses & Notes

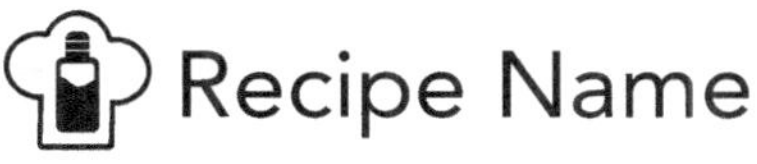 # Recipe Name

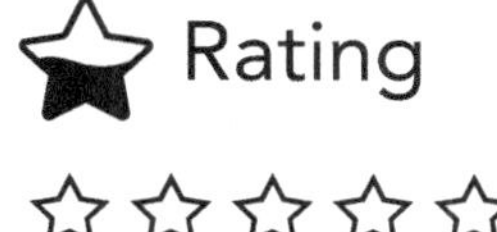
Rating

☆ ☆ ☆ ☆ ☆

Ingredients

Directions

Uses & Notes

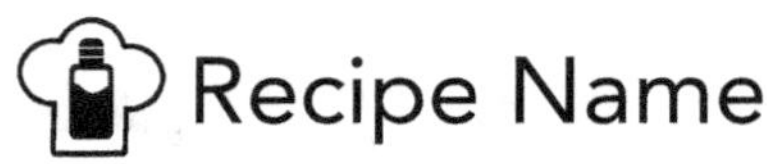 **Recipe Name**

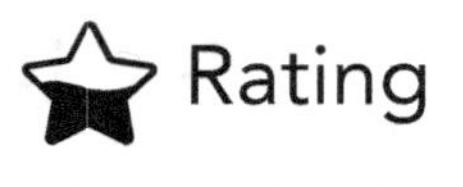 Rating
☆ ☆ ☆ ☆ ☆

Ingredients

Directions

Uses & Notes

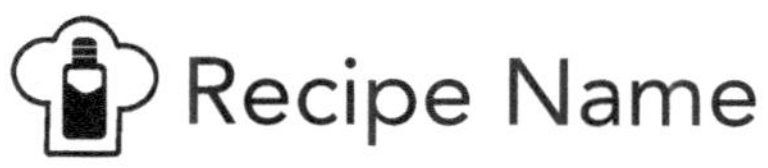 # Recipe Name

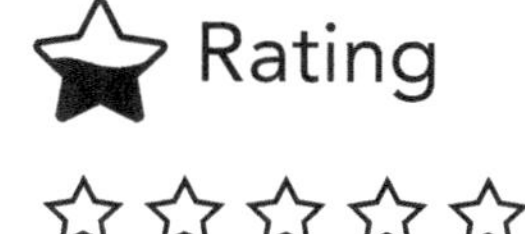 Rating

☆ ☆ ☆ ☆ ☆

Ingredients

Directions

Uses & Notes

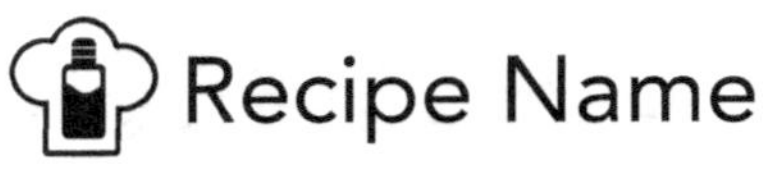 **Recipe Name**

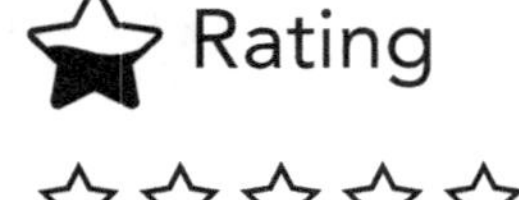 **Rating**

☆ ☆ ☆ ☆ ☆

Ingredients

Directions

Uses & Notes

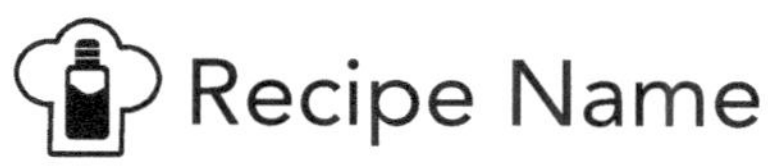

Recipe Name

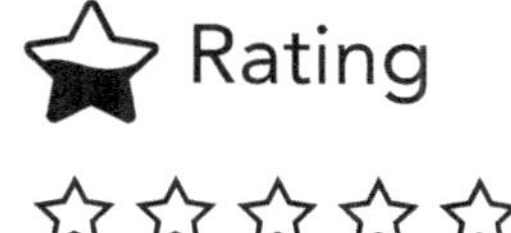

Rating
☆ ☆ ☆ ☆ ☆

Ingredients

Directions

Uses & Notes

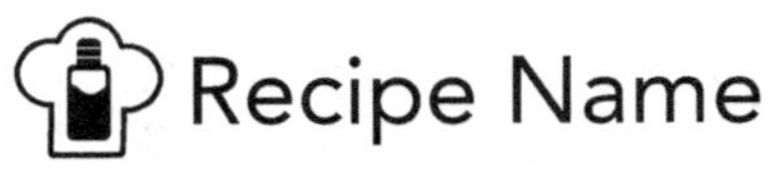 **Recipe Name**

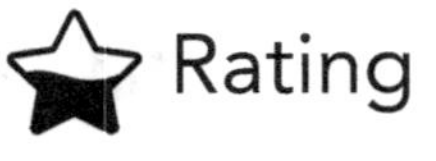 **Rating**

☆ ☆ ☆ ☆ ☆

Ingredients

Directions

Uses & Notes

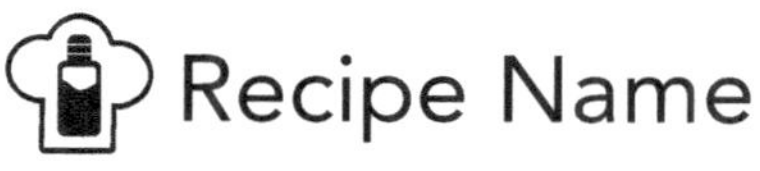 # Recipe Name

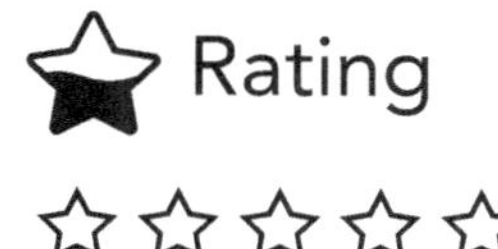 Rating

☆ ☆ ☆ ☆ ☆

Ingredients

Directions

Uses & Notes

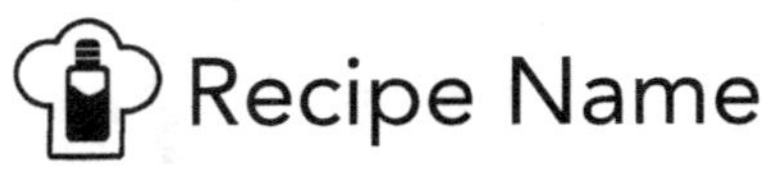 Recipe Name

Rating

☆ ☆ ☆ ☆ ☆

Ingredients

Directions

Uses & Notes

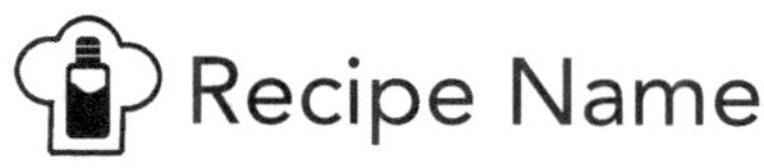 # Recipe Name

⭐ Rating
☆ ☆ ☆ ☆ ☆

Ingredients

Directions

Uses & Notes

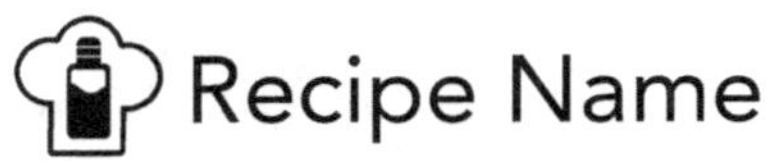 Recipe Name

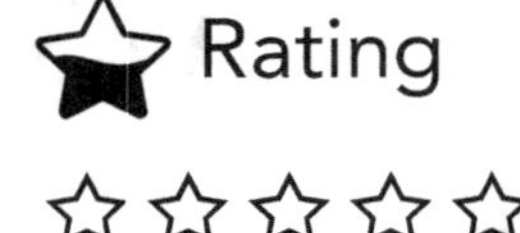 Rating

☆ ☆ ☆ ☆ ☆

Ingredients

Directions

Uses & Notes

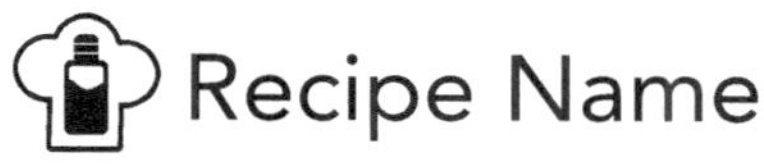 # Recipe Name

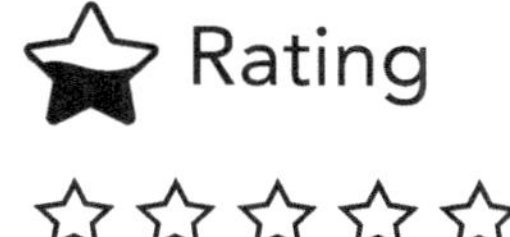 Rating

☆ ☆ ☆ ☆ ☆

Ingredients

Directions

Uses & Notes

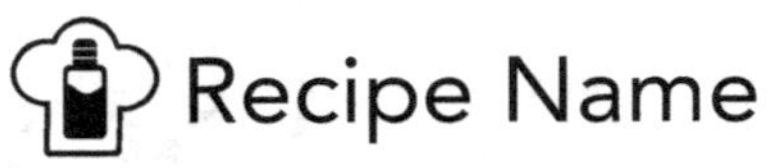 **Recipe Name**

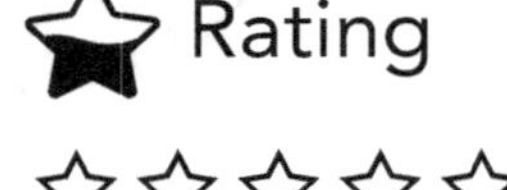 **Rating**

☆ ☆ ☆ ☆ ☆

Ingredients

Directions

Uses & Notes

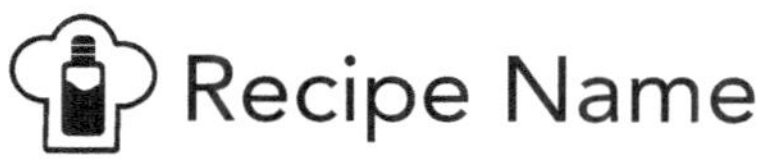 # Recipe Name

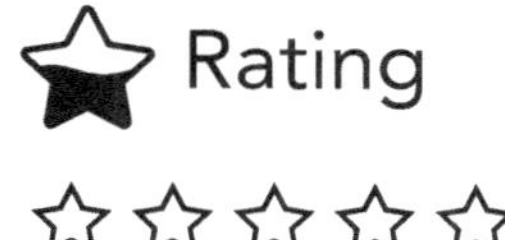 Rating

☆ ☆ ☆ ☆ ☆

Ingredients

Directions

Uses & Notes

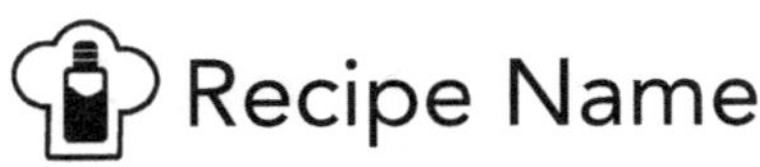 Recipe Name

Rating

☆ ☆ ☆ ☆ ☆

Ingredients

Directions

Uses & Notes

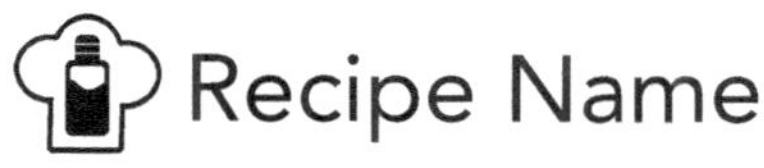# Recipe Name

☆ Rating

☆ ☆ ☆ ☆ ☆

Ingredients

Directions

Uses & Notes

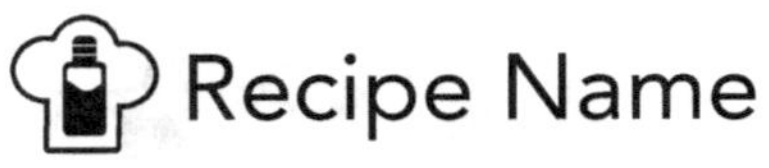 **Recipe Name**

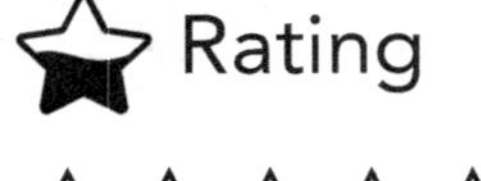 **Rating**

☆ ☆ ☆ ☆ ☆

Ingredients

Directions

Uses & Notes

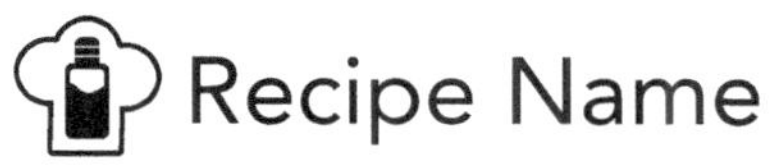 # Recipe Name

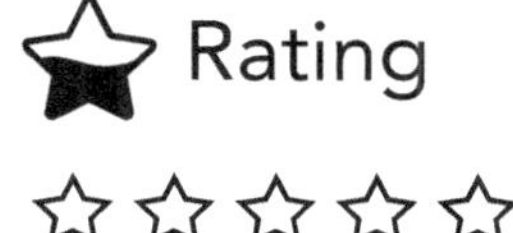 Rating
☆ ☆ ☆ ☆ ☆

Ingredients

Directions

Uses & Notes

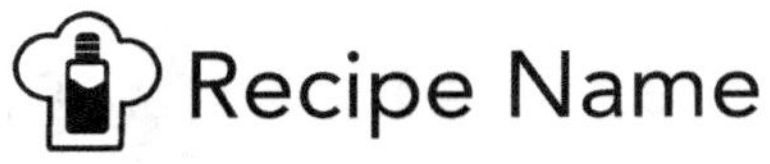 Recipe Name

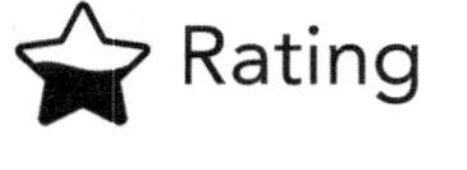 Rating
☆ ☆ ☆ ☆ ☆

Ingredients

Directions

Uses & Notes

81

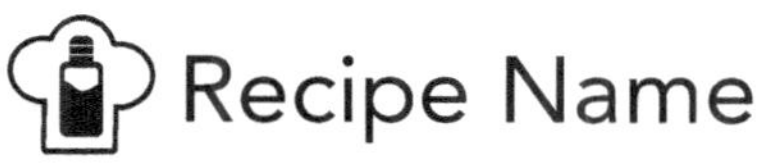 # Recipe Name

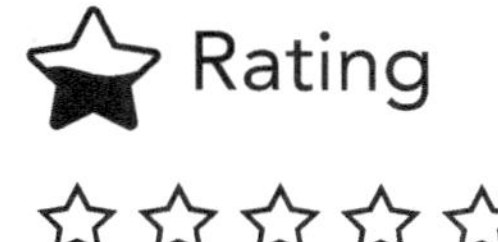 Rating
☆ ☆ ☆ ☆ ☆

Ingredients

Directions

Uses & Notes

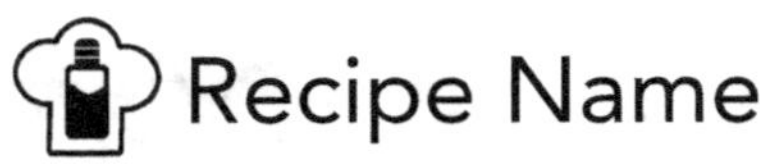 **Recipe Name**

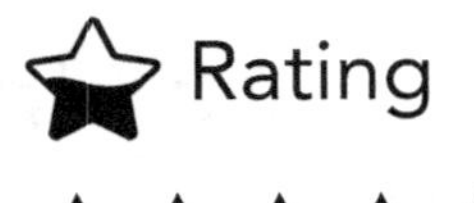 Rating

☆ ☆ ☆ ☆ ☆

Ingredients

Directions

Uses & Notes

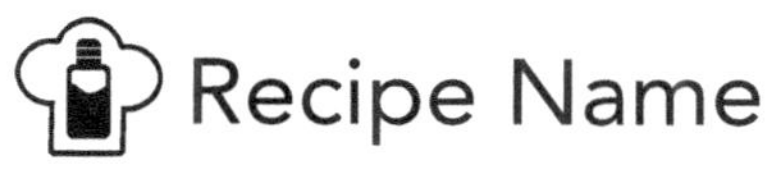 # Recipe Name

Rating
☆ ☆ ☆ ☆ ☆

Ingredients

Directions

Uses & Notes

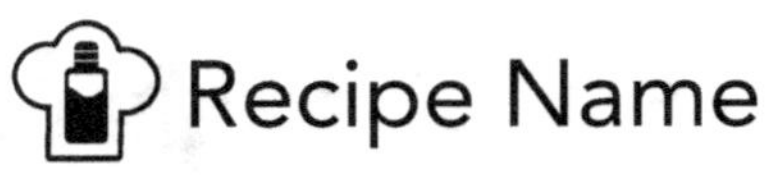 Recipe Name

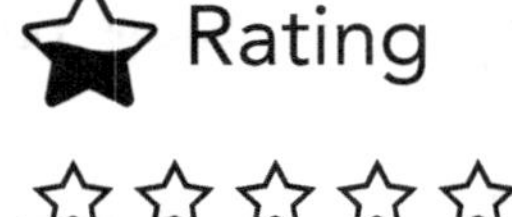 Rating

Ingredients

Directions

Uses & Notes

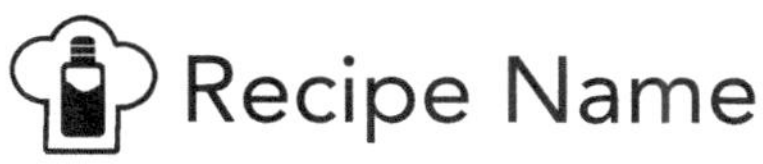 # Recipe Name

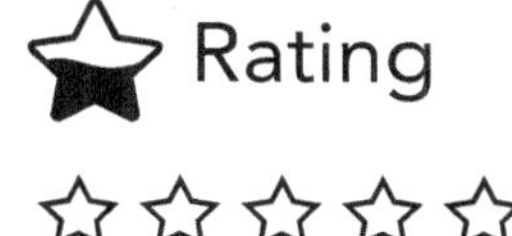 Rating
☆ ☆ ☆ ☆ ☆

Ingredients

Directions

Uses & Notes

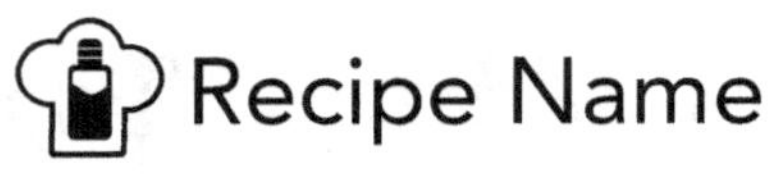 # Recipe Name

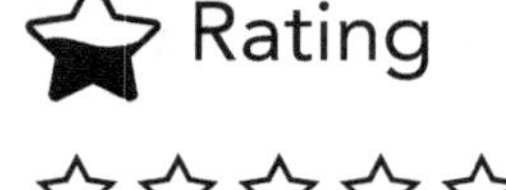 Rating

☆ ☆ ☆ ☆ ☆

Ingredients

Directions

Uses & Notes

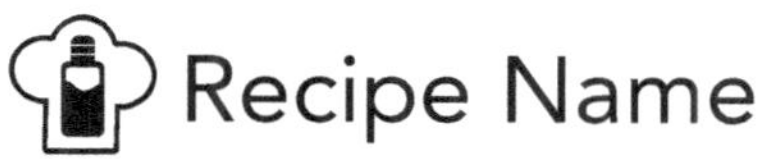 # Recipe Name

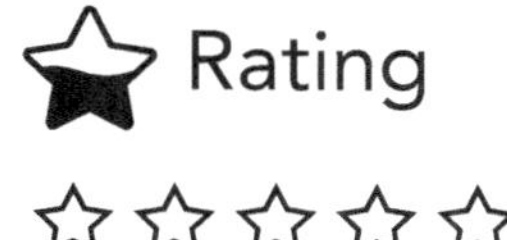 Rating

☆ ☆ ☆ ☆ ☆

Ingredients

Directions

Uses & Notes

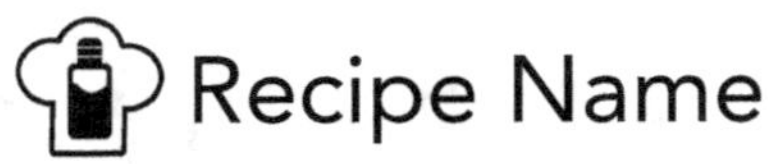 # Recipe Name

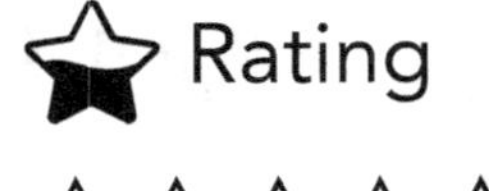 Rating
☆ ☆ ☆ ☆ ☆

Ingredients

Directions

Uses & Notes

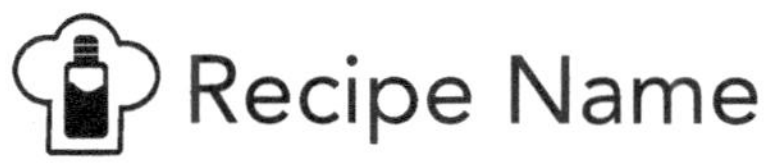 Recipe Name

Rating

☆ ☆ ☆ ☆ ☆

Ingredients

Directions

Uses & Notes

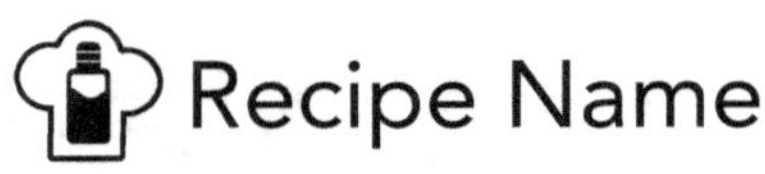 **Recipe Name**

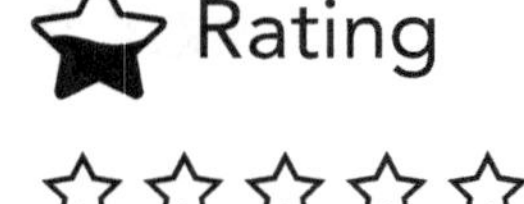 **Rating**

☆ ☆ ☆ ☆ ☆

Ingredients

Directions

Uses & Notes

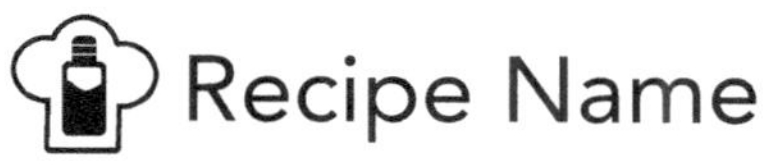 Recipe Name

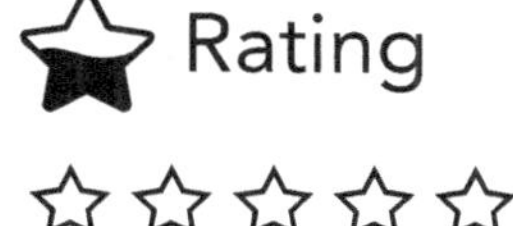 Rating

☆ ☆ ☆ ☆ ☆

Ingredients

Directions

Uses & Notes

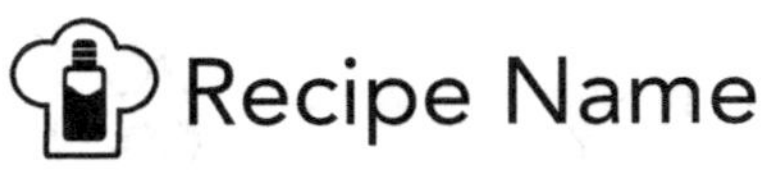 # Recipe Name

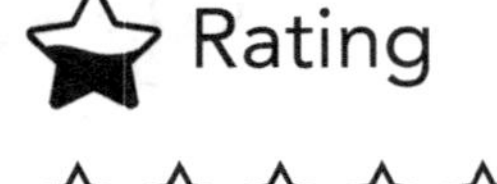 Rating

☆ ☆ ☆ ☆ ☆

Ingredients

Directions

Uses & Notes

93

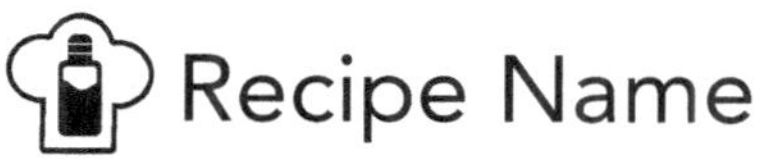 Recipe Name

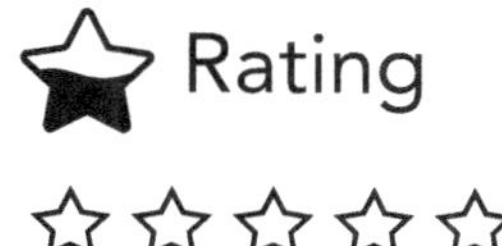 Rating

☆ ☆ ☆ ☆ ☆

Ingredients

Directions

Uses & Notes

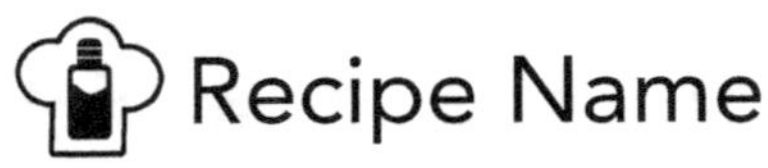 **Recipe Name**

⭐ **Rating**

☆ ☆ ☆ ☆ ☆

Ingredients

Directions

Uses & Notes

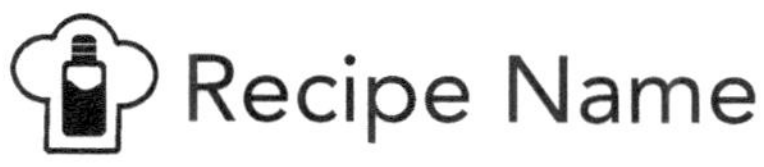 # Recipe Name

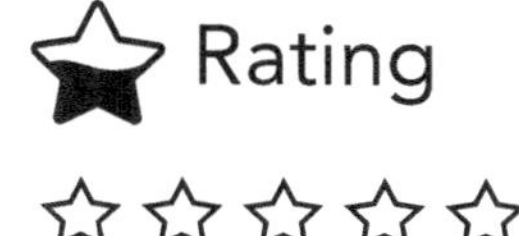 Rating
☆ ☆ ☆ ☆ ☆

Ingredients

Directions

Uses & Notes

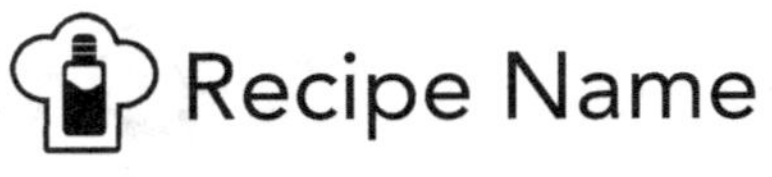 Recipe Name

Rating

☆ ☆ ☆ ☆ ☆

Ingredients

Directions

Uses & Notes

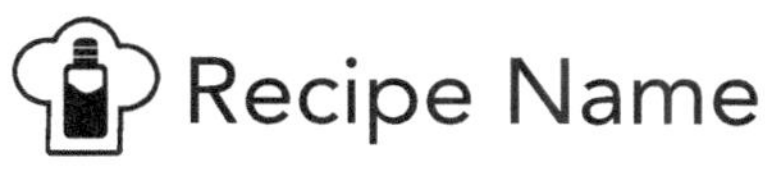 # Recipe Name

 Rating
☆ ☆ ☆ ☆ ☆

Ingredients

Directions

Uses & Notes

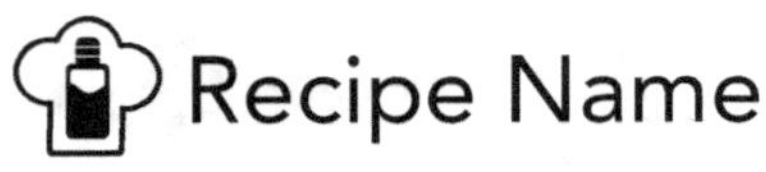 Recipe Name

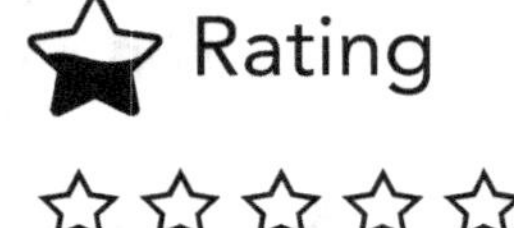 Rating

Ingredients

Directions

Uses & Notes

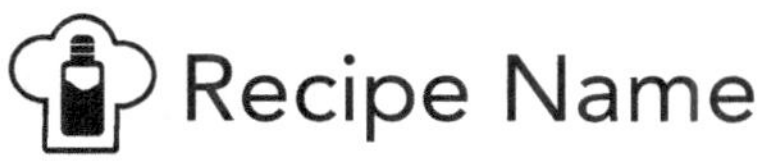 # Recipe Name

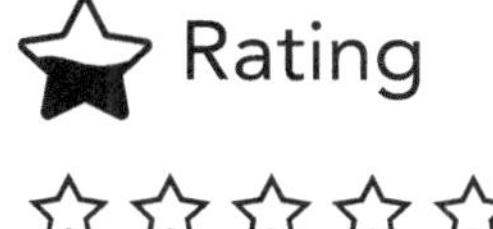 Rating

☆ ☆ ☆ ☆ ☆

Ingredients

Directions

Uses & Notes

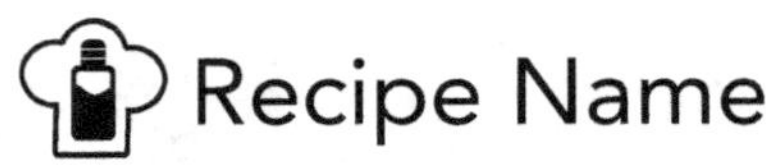 Recipe Name

⭐ Rating

☆ ☆ ☆ ☆ ☆

Ingredients

Directions

Uses & Notes

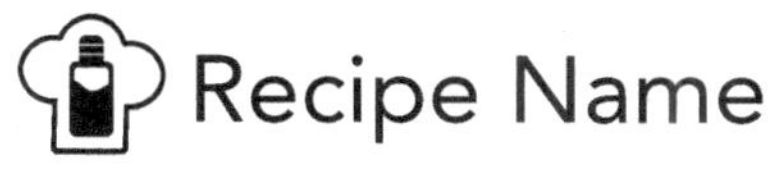 # Recipe Name

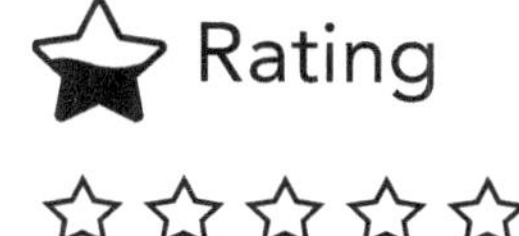 Rating

☆ ☆ ☆ ☆ ☆

Ingredients

Directions

Uses & Notes

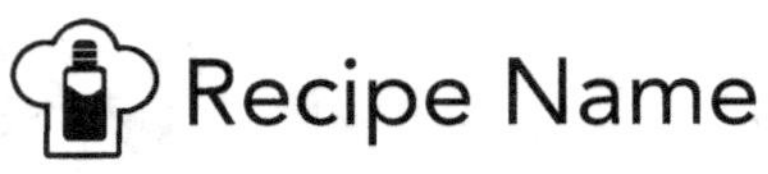 **Recipe Name**

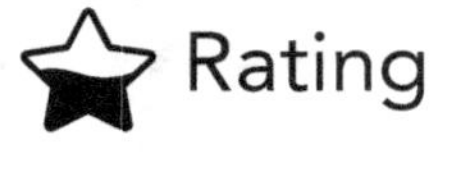 **Rating**

☆ ☆ ☆ ☆ ☆

Ingredients

Directions

Uses & Notes

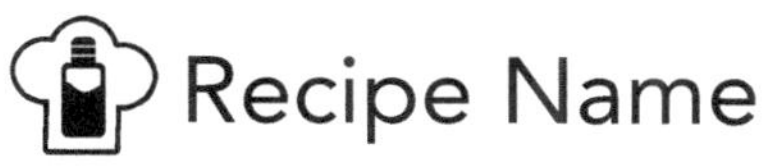 # Recipe Name

☆ Rating

☆ ☆ ☆ ☆ ☆

Ingredients

Directions

Uses & Notes

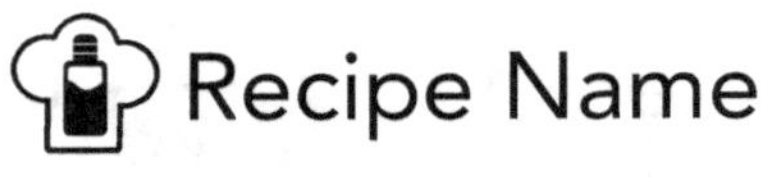 # Recipe Name

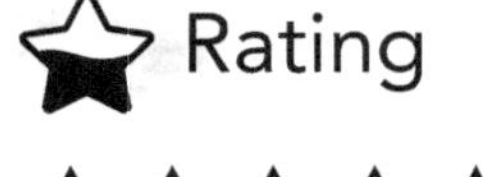 Rating

☆ ☆ ☆ ☆ ☆

Ingredients

Directions

Uses & Notes

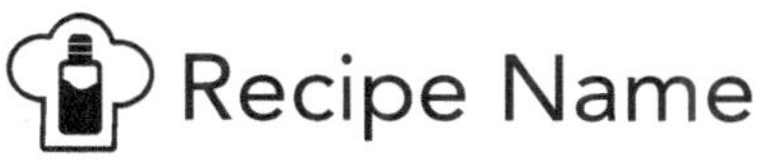 # Recipe Name

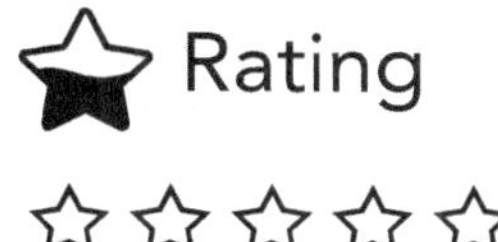 Rating

☆ ☆ ☆ ☆ ☆

Ingredients

Directions

Uses & Notes

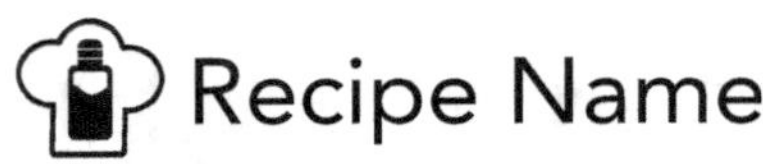 **Recipe Name**

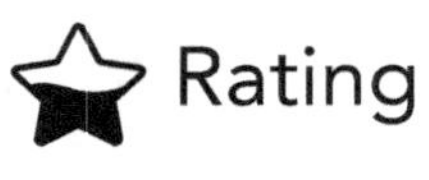 Rating
☆ ☆ ☆ ☆ ☆

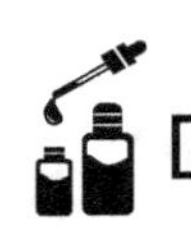 Ingredients

Directions

Uses & Notes